Autoimmune Protocol Diet:

Tips for Planning Meals for Healthy Living

Dr. Louvenia W. Williamson

TABLE OF CONTENT

- Garlic and Herb Roasted Turkey
- AIP Shepherd's Pie

Chapter 6:

Side Dishes on the Autoimmune Protocol
- Roasted Brussels Sprouts with Bacon and Apple
- Garlic and Herb Mashed Cauliflower
- Roasted Carrots with Thyme
- AIP Fried Plantains

Chapter 7:
Desserts on the Autoimmune Protocol
- Chocolate Coconut Pudding
- AIP Apple Crumble
- AIP Pumpkin Pie
- Coconut Milk Ice Cream

Chapter 8:

Tips for Sticking to the Autoimmune Protocol

- Take it back to basics
- Create rituals that works for you
- Accept that you are human
- It's not just about die
- Get some support.

CHAPTER ONE.

1.0 Introduction:

An Autoimmune Protocol (AIP) eating plan might be comparable to the paleo diet but is generally more stringent. It includes removing specific foods that may trigger inflammation and reintroducing them gradually after symptoms resolve.

The AIP diet tries to alleviate inflammation, pain, and other symptoms caused by autoimmune illnesses, such as lupus, inflammatory bowel disease (IBD), celiac disease, and rheumatoid arthritis.

Many individuals who have followed the AIP diet report improvements in their feelings and decreases in typical symptoms of autoimmune illnesses, such as tiredness and stomach or joint discomfort. Yet, although studies on this diet are intriguing, it's still restricted.

This page presents a full review of the AIP diet, including the science behind it, as well as what is presently known about its capacity to alleviate symptoms of autoimmune illnesses.

1.1 What is the Autoimmune Protocol Diet?

A healthy immune system is supposed to create antibodies that target foreign or dangerous cells in your body.

However, in persons, the immune system tends to create antibodies that, rather than combat infections, destroy healthy cells and tissues.

This may result in various symptoms, including joint discomfort, weariness, gastrointestinal pain, diarrhea, cognitive fog, and tissue and nerve damage.

Examples of autoimmune illnesses are rheumatoid arthritis, lupus, IBD, type 1 diabetes, and psoriasis.

Autoimmune illnesses are considered to be caused by a range of variables, including genetic tendency, infection, stress, inflammation, and pharmaceutical usage.

Commonly, some evidence shows that, in susceptible people, disruption to the gut barrier may lead to increased intestinal permeability, also known as "leaky gut," which may promote the development of certain autoimmune illnesses.

Certain meals may enhance the gut's permeability, raising your chance of a leaky gut.

The AIP diet focuses on removing these items and substituting them with health-promoting. These nutrient-dense foods are considered to help repair the gut and, eventually, decrease inflammation and symptoms of autoimmune illnesses.

It also eliminates some substances like gluten, which may induce aberrant immunological reactions in vulnerable people.

While scientists feel that a leaky gut may be a credible explanation for the inflammation experienced by persons with autoimmune illnesses, they caution that the existing evidence makes it hard to demonstrate a cause-and-effect link between the two.

Therefore, further study is required before firm conclusions can be drawn.

1.2 How the Autoimmune Protocol works

After the elimination phase of the diet, you reintroduce eliminated food categories one at a time and analyze your response. If a response develops, these items should be re-eliminated and retested for tolerance later (typically at least after another month of abstinence from the diet) (usually at least after another month of removal from the diet). The autoimmune protocol (AIP) diet helps to reveal a more tailored Paleo-based diet that helps to decrease inflammation, promote gut healing, and lessen autoimmune-related symptoms in the long term.

Beyond only a diet, the autoimmune protocol also stresses a way of life that prioritizes proper sleep, stress reduction, and regular physical exercise since these lifestyle variables are proven to affect autoimmunity symptoms directly. At Parsley Health, we support these self-care habits as vital components in attaining maximum health and well-being for all people.

Until recently, the autoimmune Paleo diet's efficacy was only backed by the anecdotal experiences of hundreds of individuals who successfully adopted the program to help treat and even cure their autoimmune condition. But a recent study in the last several years in both the journals Inflammatory Bowel

Disorders and Current Developments in Nutrition explored the usefulness of AIP for inflammatory bowel disease, a group of inflammatory disorders of the colon and small intestine. In both investigations, the researchers discovered that most study participants, higher than 70% in each study, attained remission after 6 weeks of following AIP. These findings add much-needed scientific backing to the autoimmune regimen and its capacity to treat patients with autoimmune illnesses.

Is the AIP Diet good for you? Is it healthy?

Following the autoimmune Paleo diet is unnecessary if you don't have an autoimmune condition. There is no reason to fear any food categories if you are generally healthy and symptom-free since the most nutritious diet is genuinely one that delivers the most range of nutrients from whole food sources.

If you've been diagnosed with an autoimmune illness and wish to manage current and continuing symptoms better, AIP might be a helpful solution. However, due to the very restricted nature of AIP, it's not recommended to attempt it if you are at risk of eating disorders, have food aversions, are hesitant to make dietary adjustments, or have other diet-related medical concerns.

If you believe the AIP diet may be too limiting for you, many members at Parsley Health typically achieve excellent results when applying less rigorous elimination diets like the Paleo diet first. If you've previously tried other kinds of elimination diets without success or a decrease in symptoms, AIP could be worth testing as a next step.

Get started with the autoimmune Paleo diet.

For the first 30-day period, you avoid dairy, gluten, grains and pseudograins, legumes, nuts, seeds, nightshade vegetables, eggs, contemporary vegetable oils, alcohol, added sugar or sweeteners, food additives, and NSAIDs. With the elimination of these suspected gut irritants, the diet focuses on including more anti-inflammatory, nutrient-dense foods such as vegetables of all kinds and colors (except nightshades), well-sourced organic meat and organ meats, wild-caught fish, fermented foods, bone broths, healthy fats from avocados, olives, and coconuts, and small amounts of antioxidant-rich fruits like berries.

While AIP may appear overwhelming and restricting, many healthful meals may be readily tweaked to meet the bill.

Some unique Parsley Health dishes you can check out if you're going AIP include:

Easy Wild Salmon Salad: To make AIP-friendly, eliminate the sundried tomatoes and add black pepper to taste.

Bison Burgers:

- Ditch the tomato slice on top.
- Go for some fresh cucumber or red onions instead.
- Miss out on dusting with black pepper.

Green Detox Smoothie: Replace the almond butter with coconut butter or avocado and exchange our Parsley Health Rebuild plant-based protein powder for some collagen peptides; you're ready to go!

How to tell whether the AIP diet worked for you

While 30 days is a recommended minimum length of time to follow the diet, it is best to wait to observe demonstrable improvement in the autoimmune disorders and accompanying symptoms before commencing reintroductions. An exclusion diet is not designed to continue forever, but it might take some individuals 30 days and others a few months to notice a substantial improvement in symptom success with AIP. Once progress is observed, you reintroduce meals safely and carefully following a structured timetable. We suggest engaging with one of our health coaches at Parsley Health for assistance when challenging and reintroducing foods. The ultimate objective of AIP is to design a tailored diet that uncovers particular food triggers and will aid healing in the long term.

For people dealing with symptoms connected to autoimmune illness like tiredness, muscle and joint discomfort, bloating, gas, rashes, hair loss, and general body pains, a decrease in these symptoms may often be a clear indicator that AIP is working. In addition to the reduction in overt physical symptoms, being tested by your doctor for changes in inflammatory markers and the health of the gut flora is the most objective approach to prove the diet has created a drop in inflammation in the body.

We have witnessed success and even total illness remission at Parsley

Health in patients with autoimmune disorders such as multiple sclerosis, eosinophilic esophagitis, systemic lupus erythematosus, and inflammatory bowel disease, among others!

One member came to us with eosinophilic esophagitis, an autoimmune reflux cause. Her ailment was fully cured with the AIP diet and a gut-healing treatment we utilize at Parsley Health.

Our takeout

AIP may be particularly beneficial for persons with a documented autoimmune illness who have attempted various dietary adjustments without a successful improvement in symptoms.

Elimination diets are generally recognized in the medical world as an effective technique for detecting food triggers.
The autoimmune Paleo diet should be considered an elimination diet focused on assessing all possibly inflammatory foods for a highly reactive population.
The autoimmune protocol is best used as a tool to help tailor the diet to include the items that help people feel their best while keeping inflammation and symptoms to a minimum. It should be followed only short term.

1.3 Benefits of following the Autoimmune Protocol.

The AIP diet may contribute to a reduction in common autoimmune disorder symptoms.
Participants reported fewer IBD-related symptoms in a study following a group of people using the AIP diet with IBD (inflammatory bowel disease). They found an improvement in stress, bowel frequency, and their ability to perform leisure and sports activities.

In another research, women with HT (Hashimoto's thyroiditis) who followed the AIP diet for 10 weeks saw a 29% drop in inflammation and a 68% reduction in disease-related symptoms after the trial.

While the study is encouraging, it's also restricted. As more AIP diet research and data surface, we may learn more about the influence of this diet.

Is the AIP diet a good choice for you?

Determining if the AIP diet is the right choice for you depends on several factors.

Firstly, knowing if it's sustainable for you and your lifestyle is essential. If enjoying food socially is a big part of your life, it might be more challenging to adopt a diet.

And although some studies support claims of the diet's positive effects, there must be a way to determine if it will work for you in advance. It's always best to consult with a healthcare professional before you make a sudden and significant change to your diet.

Conclusion

The AIP diet may help lessen symptoms of autoimmune illnesses. While some evidence supports its usefulness, it's essential to talk with a healthcare expert before adopting a new diet—especially one with many limitations.

It might be a terrific alternative if you're ready for the lifestyle transition and can stick to the diet while acquiring the nutrients required to live a healthy life.

If autoimmune symptoms are harming your quality of life, choices may be available to help improve them—the AIP diet may be one possibility.

If someone you know would benefit from this information, consider sharing it. You never know; you may help someone transform their life!

CHAPTER 2

2.0 The Basics of the Autoimmune Protocol.

No diet will heal arthritis, but can a diet relieve arthritis symptoms? Research offers the famous Mediterranean diet top marks for its anti-inflammatory advantages and diversified food options. While vegetarian and vegan diets are more restricted, studies also reveal anti-inflammatory effects.

One more restricted diet plan you may hear about is the AIP or autoimmune protocol diet. It's based on the premise that some foods inflame your gut and that avoiding them may improve autoimmune symptoms.

It's crucial to recognize that following the AIP long-term might result in nutritional shortages that can lead to various issues. Plus, there needs to be a clear, organized strategy, so assessing whether a modified version would be ideal for your circumstances is challenging.

2.1 Foods to avoid on the Autoimmune Protocol

Below are the foods to avoid on the Autoimmune protocol:

- Grains

- Dairy
- Eggs
- Trans Fats
- Chemical Additives
- Artificial Flavorings
- High-Fructose
- Corn Syrup
- Legumes & Beans
- Soy
- Nuts
- Processed Foods
- Seeds
- Vegetable Oils
- Night Shades
- Alcohol
- Coffee

The food categories to avoid on the AIP diet are considered to promote gut permeability, which may cause harm to the gut barrier. This may lead to issues such as a "leaky gut," which may be a trigger for symptoms in persons with autoimmune illnesses. People with IBS or IBD, especially Crohn's Disease, may also have inflammation and digestive difficulties while ingesting certain foods.

2.2 Foods to include in the Autoimmune Protocol

It is suggested to eat the items listed on the Autoimmune protocol:

- Meat
- Fish
- Vegetables (excluding Night Shades

- Sweet Potatoes
- Fruit (small amounts)
- Avocado Oil
- Coconut Oil
- Olive Oil
- Coconut Milk
- Dairy-Free Fermented Foods
- Honey or Maple Syrup
- Broth
- Vinegars

Nutrient-dense meals like these are high in vitamins and other nutrients, which may help lessen symptoms of autoimmune illnesses. The AIP encourages the intake and preparation of fresh, nutrient-dense meals, bone broth, good fats, fatty fish, shellfish, fermented foods, and organic vegetables and fresh fruit —

as long as they're not on the AIP exclusion list.

2.3 How to convert to the Autoimmune Protocol

My top recommendations get you to prepare correctly for the elimination phase by making it simpler to smoothly transition into the protocol with a better probability of success adhering to it.

First, know what's prohibited and included in the AIP diet.

Here is a short glance at the meals you will eliminate:
- Chocolate
- Coffee

- Dairy
- Eggs
- Fruit-based spices (such black pepper and nutmeg)
- Gluten
- Grains
- Gums and additives
- Legumes / Beans
- Nightshade vegetables and spices (including cayenne, tomatoes, and eggplant)
- Nuts
- Industrialized, GMO cooking oils (corn, soy, sunflower, vegetable oils, etc.) (corn, soy, sunflower, vegetable oils, etc.)
- Processed, refined, and fast foods
- Pseudogrians (quinoa, millet, amaranth, etc.) (quinoa, millet, amaranth, etc.)

- Refined sugar
- Seeds Spices including nightshades and seeds
- Soy

Here are some of the dishes you will be eating:

- Bone broth
- Clean proteins (eg, wild-caught fish; pastured hog, chicken, cattle, and offal)
- Collagen
- Cultured foods
- Healthy fats
- Herbal teas
- Lots of vegetables
- Nourishing soups

Track Your Current Diet, then Eliminate Gradually.

Before you shift to the AIP elimination phase, taking stock of what you presently consume might be incredibly useful. This helps since you know what items you presently consume that are acceptable on the AIP diet and highlight what areas you struggle with the most.

If you notice that you are eating cheese at nearly every meal, you may want the cheese to be the final food group.

By the way, this non-fortified nutritional yeast offers an AIP-compliant cheesy taste to your recipes without dairy!

While a few individuals do great with the "cold turkey" approach when going from a typical American diet to the AIP elimination phase, this is generally not the case for most other people.

You could be better off with a more gradual adjustment. This might imply converting only one meal or snack daily from your present diet to the AIP diet. This might also mean removing one of the "no" items every week or every few days until your diet is entirely elimination compliant. At this moment, when you are respectful, you will begin your 30 days of 100% AIP.

An example of this would be to swap the burger and fries you eat once a week for a bunless burger topped with sliced cucumber, mango, and lettuce, then served with sweet potato chips which have been fried in coconut oil. This would be a fantastic dinner exchange!

Another example would be to swap the low-fat milk you drink in your morning tea to additive-free coconut milk, or if you are allergic to coconut, you may use my homemade tiger nut milk recipe. This would be an ingredient exchange!

If you currently consume a decent quantity of foods permitted on the AIP, you can switch to it more quickly. Those who have been on a Paleo diet for a few months before starting the AIP are likely to have a greater success rate of shifting rapidly into the AIP. This is because a Paleo diet is already devoid of gluten, dairy, grains, legumes, and harmful food-like compounds in fast food and processed supermarket goods.

2.4 Tips for meal planning on the Autoimmune Protocol

Tips to Keep in Mind during AIP Meal Planning

- For starters, make sure your meals fit your timetable. If you're busy, plan meals that are fast and simple to make.
- Try to make meals that will offer you lunch leftovers for the following day.
- If snacks are a necessity, opt for no-prep.

AIP Meal Planning Suggestions

These meal choices are targeted toward offering you ideas and inspiration as you follow your meal-planning adventure. As you begin researching your recipes, you'll quickly learn there are many beautiful things to select from. To make your search much more straightforward, try utilizing our Real Plans app. It will help you choose and choose meals that will fit you and your family's lifestyle.

Breakfast Ideas:

- Apple Berry Smoothie
- Sweet Potato Bowl
- Strawberry Banana Acai Smoothie

Lunch Ideas:

- Egg Roll in a Bowl
- Avocado Tuna Salad
- Lemon-Fried Avocado
- Chicken Sage Hash
- Chicken Avocado Soup
- Southwest Salad with Pork

Dinner Ideas:

- One-Pan Chicken Pesto
- Unstuffed Cabbage Roll
- Ground Beef Stir Fry
- Instant Pot Beef Brisket

Snack Ideas:

- Sliced Cucumbers
- Diced Roasted Acorn Squash
- Berries

CHAPTER THREE

3.0 Breakfast Recipes on the Autoimmune Protocol

The morning could be a busy and chaotic time, but the last thing I want to do is miss breakfast. Since maintaining my blood sugar level has been critical in controlling my various autoimmune disorders, it's the day's most important meal! I make sure that I fit in something every morning so I can stay feeling my best.

The following Quick & Easy AIP Breakfast options are favorable for an AIP diet and incredibly quick to put together! Plus, they are gluten-free, grain-free, refined sugar-free, and dairy-free. Some of these may even be prepared the night before. Check them out to liven up your anti-inflammatory morning.

3.1 Sweet Potato Breakfast Bowl

This Sweet Potato Breakfast Bowl is the ultimate egg and grain-free breakfast! It has the sensation of eating oatmeal but is created with components like sweet potato and coconut milk rather than Grain.

There's something so warm and cozy about a big breakfast bowl. Oatmeal is a typical breakfast option for many, but if you're grain-free, you wind up losing out on this traditional breakfast. This sweet potato breakfast bowl is a creative grain-free variation that combines mashed sweet potato, coconut milk, and any toppings of your choosing!

THE INGREDIENTS FOR THE SWEET POTATO BREAKFAST BOWL

- Sweet potato.
- Coconut milk. I like the brand, Native Forest.
- Toppings of your choosing. I used coconut yogurt, almond butter, blueberries, slivered almonds, and cinnamon.

HOW TO MAKE A SWEET POTATO BREAKFAST BOWL

- Bake the sweet potato. Preheat the oven and bake in the oven for around an hour or until tender.
- Mash the sweet potato. Scoop out the sweet potato and discard the skin. Mash with coconut milk and salt. \s* Add toppings & serve. Top the mashed sweet potato with coconut yogurt, almond butter, almonds, blueberries, and cinnamon. Serve heated with a spoon.

WHAT OTHER TOPPINGS CAN YOU ADD TO THE BREAKFAST BOWL?

- Grain-free granola
- Diced apples
- Raisins

- Pomegranate seeds
- Nut or seed butter of your choice \s*
- Tigernut butter
- Shredded coconut Etc!

CAN YOU MAKE THIS BREAKFAST BOWL AHEAD OF TIME?

You can roast the sweet potato ahead of time and prepare the toppings when you're ready to serve it!

HOW CAN YOU ADD EXTRA PROTEIN TO THIS BREAKFAST BOWL?

You can add a protein powder to the sweet potato as you mash it!

3.2 AIP Breakfast Hash

This well-rounded meal skips eggs in favor of herb-seasoned sausage, veggies, and a side of seasonal fruit for an AIP Friendly breakfast that satisfies. Ground pork may be replaced with ground turkey, chicken, or beef.

AIP-Friendly Breakfast Hash Ingredients:

- 2 tbsp olive oil
- 3 cups peeled/sliced sweet potatoes
- 1 lb. brussels sprouts, halved

- 2 cups chopped kale
- 1 lb. ground pork
- 1 tbsp Paleo Powder AIP Seasoning
- For Serving
- 2 cups fresh cherries
- 2 cups diced pineapple

AIP Friendly Breakfast Hash

This well-rounded meal skips eggs in favor of herb-seasoned sausage, veggies, and a side of seasonal fruit for an AIP Friendly breakfast that satisfies. Ground pork may be replaced with ground turkey, chicken, or beef.

Course Breakfast, brunch Cuisine American Keyword AIP,

AIP Friendly, breakfast, brunch, gluten-free, paleo, Pork, whole30

- Prep Time 10 minutes
- Cook Time 27 minutes
- Total Time 37 minutes
- Servings 4 meals
- Calories 530kcal
- Author Meal Prep on Fleek

Ingredients
- 2 tbsp olive oil
- 3 cups peeled/sliced sweet potatoes
- 1 lb. brussels sprouts halved
- 2 cups chopped kale
- 1 lb. mince pork
- 1 tbsp Paleo Powder AIP Seasoning
- For Serving

- 2 cups fresh cherries
- 2 cups diced pineapple

Instructions

- Heat olive oil over medium-high heat in a big heavy pan or Dutch oven. Add sweet potatoes and Brussels sprouts and sauté for 10 minutes covered, stirring periodically.

- Move sweet potatoes and Brussels sprouts to one side and add meat to the pan. Use a spatula to split Pork up into tiny bits. Brown for 5 minutes. Sprinkle Paleo Powder Seasoning over beef and veggies and mix thoroughly.

Cook 7-10 minutes longer, uncovered, until meat is cooked through and sweet potatoes are soft. Stir in kale and simmer for 2 minutes to wilt.

- Divide hash into significant divisions of 4 MPOF teal containers and add cherries and pineapple to the little compartments. Refrigerate until serving.

3.3 Blueberry Coconut Smoothie Bowl

This nutritious, low-sugar blueberry coconut smoothie bowl tastes like blueberry ice cream but won't spike your blood sugar and will help keep you full and invigorate you for hours.

COCONUT HEALTH BENEFITS

You could prepare this smoothie using fresh coconut flesh, but not everyone can acquire it in their region, so today, we're going to use unsweetened shredded coconut. If you can get your hands on fresh coconut, go for it. I can generally locate new coconut flesh at my local Whole Foods Market, and I'll frequently buy up a container and freeze it for smoothies. Fresh coconut in this smoothie is incredible, but for today, we'll make it accessible with unsweetened shredded coconut.

WHAT ARE MCTS?

Unsweetened shredded coconut still provides many health advantages, so feel free to lose out if you can't locate fresh coconut. While shredded coconut is constituted nearly entirely of fat, virtually all of which is saturated fat in the form of MCTs or medium-chain triglycerides, shredded coconut is nevertheless linked with several health advantages.

MCTs have been demonstrated to raise HDL cholesterol, offer a quick energy source, promote satiety, and accelerate metabolism. In addition, the MCTs contained in coconut, lauric, caprylic, and capric acid all have antibacterial, antiviral, and anti-fungal qualities, which is why coconut oil is so helpful in and out of the kitchen.

COCONUT NUTRITION

Coconut is also a tasty and healthy source of fiber, vitamins, minerals, and amino acids, including calcium, potassium, and magnesium. Coconut also includes a ton of electrolytes, which is why coconut water is a terrific exercise drink.

STABILIZING BLOOD SUGAR

I'm beginning to realize that stable blood sugar is vital for my health and welfare. I spoke a lot about this in my piece on controlling hunger. So, how to maintain blood sugar levels stable? The principles of keeping blood sugar levels consistent are the same as the foundations of a good diet. Let's have a look.

TIPS FOR HEALTHY BLOOD SUGAR LEVELS

- Avoid sugar and refined carbohydrates
- Include protein in every meal
- Eat low on the glycemic index (vegetables, legumes, nuts, seeds, berries, etc.)
- Include a snack between meals to prevent low blood sugar
- Ditch artificial sweeteners
- Eat whole grains instead of refined grains
- Exercise daily

- Eat a balanced breakfast
- Eat more fiber
- Manage stress levels
- Get enough sleep

HOW DOES FAT HELP BLOOD SUGAR LEVELS?

In summary, healthy fats from foods like nuts, seeds, avocado, and coconut take longer to digest, which helps our body decrease the absorption of the sugars present in carbs. Fats also don't create spike insulin which helps maintain consistent insulin levels, i.e., stable blood sugar levels. Moderating carbs and incorporating healthy fats in the diet may aid with sugar cravings, digestive difficulties, controlling blood sugar, boosting energy and sleep quality, and assisting with weight reduction.

Fat is especially effective when coupled with carbs to aid in decreasing digestion. Fats help us remain satisfied longer, reduce sugar crashes, and healthy, plant-based fats include a spectrum of potent antioxidants, vitamins, and minerals vital to optimal health. Don't be frightened of fat if you want to maintain good blood sugar levels!

BLUEBERRY HEALTH BENEFITS

We spoke about the finest superfoods to add to smoothies, and although blueberries weren't on that list, they're an everyday super-powered superfood you should undoubtedly incorporate into your diet. Blueberries are one of the most antioxidant-rich foods there are. Packed with antioxidants, vitamins, and minerals and low in sugar, they're a must-have in a healthy, well-rounded diet.

Blueberries include anthocyanins, iron, phospfibers, fiber, calcium, magnesium, manganese, zinc, and vitamin K, all of which contribute to blueberries cancer-fighting, bone-building, heart-protecting, digestive-supporting, and anti-aging properties.

This blueberry coconut smoothie bowl is a serious candidate for my fave smoothie bowl ever. It tastes like blueberry ice cream, and the texture is excellent. It is made with frozen cauliflower, zucchini, and blueberries and is incredibly low in sugar and rich in vitamins and fiber.

If you adore smoothie bowls, I'd suggest adding cutting and freezing zucchini and cauliflower to your weekly meal prep. They're the best veggies to add to smoothies since they offer plenty of volume and nutrients without affecting the taste. They also combine well when frozen to give the ideal smoothie bowl consistency.

I topped my smoothie bowl with coconut, cashews, cacao nibs, blueberries, and sunflower seed butter, but any smoothie bowl toppings work! Try your favorite chopped nuts, dried fruit, sliced banana or berries, peanut butter, tahini, hemp seeds, chia seeds, chia seed jam, and the perfect smoothie bowl topper.

3.4 Chicken Apple Breakfast Sausage Ingredients

Chicken, Dried Apples, Water. Contains Less Than 2% Of The Following: Honey, Salt, Spices, and Parsley.

Spices

Allspice, Basil, Black Pepper, Cinnamon, Parsley, Tarragon, Red Pepper

Cooking Instructions

Skillet (Preferred): Place frozen patties into a prepared pan over medium heat, rotating periodically, for 4-5 minutes.

Microwave: Place frozen patties on a paper towel on a microwave-safe dish. Do not cover. Set the microwave to medium-high (high heat toughens patties) (high heat hardens patties). Heat as follows: 2 Patties: 2-1/2 min. 4 Patties: 4 min. 6 Patties: 5-1/2 min.

CHAPTER FOUR

4.0 Snacks & Appetizers on the Autoimmune Protocol

An appetizer is a little piece of food served before the main meal, meant to whet one's appetite in anticipation of what is following.

A snack is a little piece of food consumed in-between meals, or occasionally, instead of a meal, meant to dull one's appetite until a complete meal can be taken.

The difference is not in the meal itself but in when and why it is being eaten. Anything you offer as an appetizer could be consumed as a snack.

4.1 Carrot Fries with Lemon Thyme Dip

Ingredients Dip:
- 1 cup sour cream
- 1/3 cup chopped fresh mint
- 1 1/2 teaspoons fresh lemon juice
- 2 teaspoons sugar
- 1/8 teaspoon kosher salt
- 1/8 teaspoon freshly ground black pepper

Fries:
- 5 cups safflower or vegetable oil
- 6 big egg whites, beaten

- 3 cups panko breadcrumbs (Japanese breadcrumbs) (Japanese breadcrumbs)
- 4 big carrots, peeled and sliced into 3-inch long sticks, each approximately 1/2-inch thick
- 4 big carrots, peeled and cut into 3-inch long bars, each approximately 1/2-inch thick
- Kosher salt and freshly ground black pepper for sprinkling

Directions:

- **For the dip**: In a medium bowl, whisk the sour cream, mint, lemon juice, sugar, salt, and pepper together until mixed. Cover and chill for at least 30 minutes and up to 1 day.

- **For the fries**: In a large heavy-bottomed saucepan, heat the oil over medium heat until a deep-frying thermometer registers 350 degrees F. (If you don't have a thermometer, a cube of bread will brown in approximately 3 minutes.)\

- Place the egg whites in a medium basin. Place the panko breadcrumbs in another medium bowl. Place the carrot sticks into the egg whites in batches and flip to coat. Remove the carrot sticks, letting any extra egg white fall into the dish. Drop the carrot sticks in the panko; toss lightly to cover.

- Working in batches, fry the carrot sticks until deep brown,

3 to 4 minutes, flipping and separating with a wooden spoon and adjusting the temperature to maintain 350 degrees F. Drain on paper towels.

- Place a bowl of the dip in the middle of a dish. Sprinkle the fries with salt and pepper. Arrange the fries around the drop, and serve.

4.2 AIP Guacamole

This AIP Guacamole is a nightshade-free variation of the original! It's paleo, Whole30, AIP, and simple to cook at home in just a few minutes.

What is nightshade-free guacamole? It's just the guacamole that we all know and love without tomatoes or peppers to make it AIP-compatible! I know it's extra…but it's worth it.

Everyone has their favorite guacamole, whether from a restaurant they adore or from mama's kitchen. Still, each classic version comprises a few mainstays like avocado (of course), lime juice, onions, some chilies for spice, and perhaps even some fresh garlic and cilantro. This AIP version keeps things extremely basic, using avocado, red Onion, fresh cilantro, lime juice, and other spices. Throw this up for your next taco night or party, and I promise no one will notice the nightshades!

INGREDIENTS FOR EASY AIP GUACAMOLE

- Avocado. You'll need one huge avocado or 2 tiny ones for this dish. I suggest getting your avocados at least a couple of days before you want to prepare this to ensure that they're at their optimal freshness.
- Pro tip: aim for avocados with less glossy skin and a little bit of give when you softly squeeze it with your fingertips.
- Red Onion.
- Cilantro. I know some cilantro haters out there, but this

balances out the taste of this guac.

- Lime juice. You may use juice from fresh lime or 100% organic lime juice purchased from the supermarket (ensure it doesn't have any concentrate or additives). I particularly adore Santa Cruz Organic lime juice.
- Seasonings. A little garlic, onion powder, and salt polish this guac wonderfully.

HOW TO MAKE EASY AIP GUACAMOLE

- Mash the avocado. Cut and peel the avocado into a mixing basin and mash thoroughly with a fork.

- Fold in ingredients. Add the red Onion, cilantro, lime juice, and spices and toss together.
- Serve + enjoy! Serve with your favorite grain-free chips (plantain chips are a fantastic alternative for AIP!

WHAT'S THE BEST WAY TO STORE GUACAMOLE?

Of course, guacamole is the finest fresh, but if you're preparing it ahead of time and taking it with you, here are my tips…

- Wrap it airtight. More excellent air equals more oxidation.
- Store it with the pit. If I'm keeping it for later, I put the avocado pit in the middle of the

guacamole. This truly does help keep it fresh.

- Add additional lime juice. I add more lime juice to the top to prevent it from browning.

WHAT SHOULD YOU SERVE WITH THIS GUACAMOLE?

- Plantain chips. Artisan Tropic is my fav, or try this at-home recipe here!
- Siete tortilla chips. For a grain-free chip (non-AIP).
- Sliced vegetables. Carrots, celery, and cucumber all work beautifully with this guacamole and offer a lot of extra freshness.

4.3 Coconut Bacon

If you've ever desired bacon but wanted something other than the actual thing, coconut bacon is the solution!

This dish is easy, needing only 8 ingredients, 1 skillet, and 15 minutes to cook. The result is crunchy, bacon-flavored coconut flakes that are excellent for adding to items like salads, sandwiches, dips, and more!

We hope you enjoy this recipe! If you attempt it, post a picture #minimalistbaker on Instagram, and leave a comment and rating! Thanks for supporting Minimalist Baker!

How to Make Coconut Bacon

Savory, crispy coconut bacon prepared on 1 pan in 15 minutes! Perfect for topping salads, adding to sandwiches (hello vegan BLT), dips, and more!

PREP TIME
2 minutes
COOK TIME
13 minutes
TOTAL TIME
15 minutes
Servings (1/4 cup servings)
Course Side, Snack

Cuisine Gluten-Free, Vegan
Freezer Friendly 1 month
Does it keep?
1 Week

Ingredients

- 2 cups big flake unsweetened coconut
- 1 Tbsp avocado or grapeseed oil (or similar neutral oil) (or another neutral oil)
- 2 Tbsp tamari (ensure gluten-free for GF eaters)
- 1 tsp smoky paprika
- 1 Tbsp maple syrup
- 1/2 tsp liquid smoke
- 1 sprinkle sea salt
- 1/2 tsp black pepper

Instructions

1. Preheat the oven to 325 degrees F (162 C) and line a baking sheet with parchment paper (or multiple baking sheets if increasing batch size) (or more baking sheets if increasing batch size).

2. Add coconut flake, oil, tamari, paprika, maple syrup, liquid smoke, sea salt, and black pepper. Toss/stir to thoroughly coat.

3. Bake at 325 for 6 minutes, then go and rotate the pan around. Bake for another 5-7 minutes or until coconut bacon is crispy and golden brown. Observe in

the final minutes of cooking and be cautious not to burn as it may move from brown to scorched very quickly.

4. Let cool for 10 minutes - it will continue crisping as it cools. Coconut bacon is fantastic for adding to items like salads, sandwiches, dips, and more! Store leftovers covered at room temperature for up to 1 week (occasionally longer) or in the freezer for 1 month

4.4 Sweet Potato Bites with Avocado and Bacon

Ingredients

- 2 tbsp olive oil
- 2 sweet potatoes, scrubbed clean, peels on
- 1 ¼ tsp salt, divided
- ¾ tsp pepper
- 1/3 cup sharp cheddar cheese
- 2 medium avocados, peeled, pitted and diced
- 2 tbsp nonfat or 2% Greek yogurt
- 1 tbsp fresh lime juice
- ½ tsp smoked paprika
- 3 oz bacon (about 4 slices)
- 3 tbsp freshly chopped cilantro

Directions

Place the rack in top and bottom thirds of your oven and preheat the oven to 425 degrees F. Line two rimmed baking sheets with foil, then brush each with ½ tbsp olive oil. Slice potatoes into ½ to ¼ inch cross-sections.

Arrange slices in a single layer on the greased baking pans, then brush tops with remaining olive oil. Sprinkle 1 tsp salt and black pepper. Roast for 20-25 minutes, until golden brown beneath, turning the pans 180 degrees and changing their location on the upper/lower racks halfway through. Flip and then roast for a further 8 minutes. Remove from the oven, sprinkle with cheddar, then return to the oven and bake for an additional 3 minutes until the cheese is melted and bubbling.

Meanwhile, in a separate dish, mix the avocado, Greek yogurt, lime juice, remaining 1/5 tsp salt, and smoked paprika, Mash gently with a fork, but still, leave the mixture somewhat lumpy. Set aside.

Fry bacon in a large skillet over medium heat, then remove from the pan and lay between two paper towels on a dinner plate. Blot away excess oil and slice into tiny pieces when cool enough to handle.
Once the crisps have cooked, top each with a dollop of the avocado mixture, diced bacon, and cilantro. Serve heated or at room temperature.
Yield: Makes roughly 40 bites

Nutritional Information Per Serving

- Calories: 44
- Fat: 3 g.
- Sat. Fat: 1 g.
- Trans Fat: 0 g.
- Sodium: 118 mg
- Carbs: 2 g.
- Fiber: 1 g.

CHAPTER FIVE

5.0 Main Dishes on the Autoimmune Protocol

The Autoimmune Protocol (AIP) is a specific diet to decrease inflammation and promote healing in persons with autoimmune diseases. It entails removing some foods known to induce inflammation and autoimmune responses and emphasizing nutrient-dense whole foods.

Regarding significant courses on the AIP, numerous alternatives may be both tasty and healthful.

5.1 Slow Cooker Beef Stew

Sure, I can offer you a recipe for Slow Cooker Beef Stew. Here's one:

Ingredients:

- 2 lbs beef stew meat, cut into 1-inch cubes
- 1/4 cup all-purpose flour
- 1 tsp salt
- 1/2 tsp black pepper
- 1 tsp garlic powder
- 2 tbsp vegetable oil
- 1 cup chopped onion
- 2 cloves garlic, minced
- 2 cups beef broth
- 1 cup red wine (optional)
- 1 tbsp tomato paste
- 1 tsp dried thyme
- 1 tsp dried rosemary

- 4 cups chopped vegetables (carrots, potatoes, celery)
- 1 cup frozen peas

Directions:

1. Whisk together the flour, salt, black pepper, and garlic powder in a large basin. Add the beef stew meat and stir to coat evenly.
2. Heat the vegetable oil over medium-high heat in a large skillet. Add the beef stew meat and brown on both sides, approximately 5-7 minutes. Transfer the beef to the slow cooker.
3. In the same pan, add the Onion, garlic, and sauté until soft,

approximately 5 minutes. Add the beef broth and red wine (if using), and mix to blend.

4. Add the tomato paste, thyme, and rosemary to the skillet, and mix to incorporate. Pour the mixture over the steak into the slow cooker.

5. Add the chopped veggies to the slow cooker, and stir to mix.

6. Cover the slow cooker and simmer on low for 8 hours.

7. In the final 30 minutes of simmering, add the frozen peas and mix to incorporate.

8. Serve hot, and enjoy!

Note: You may modify the veggies and spices to your desire. This recipe produces around 6 servings.

5.2 Lemon Herb Chicken Skewers

Lemon herb chicken skewers are a tasty and easy-to-make dish that's excellent for a fast weekday supper or a weekend BBQ. Here's a simple method that you can follow to create these delectable skewers:

Ingredients:

- 2 boneless, skinless chicken breasts, cut into 1-inch cubes
- 1/4 cup olive oil
- 2 tablespoons freshly squeezed lemon juice
- 2 cloves garlic, minced

- 1 tablespoon chopped fresh rosemary
- 1 tablespoon chopped new thyme
- 1/2 teaspoon salt
- 1/4 teaspoon black pepper
- Wooden skewers, soaked in water for 30 minutes

Instructions:

1. Mix the olive oil, lemon juice, garlic, rosemary, thyme, salt, and black pepper in a medium bowl.
2. Add the chicken to the bowl and toss to coat it with the marinade. Cover the bowl and refrigerate for at least 30 minutes (up to 2 hours) (or up to 2 hours).

3. Preheat a grill or grill pan over medium-high heat.
4. Thread the chicken onto the wooden skewers, spreading the chicken equally among the skewers.
5. Grill the skewers, regularly rotating, for approximately 10-12 minutes or until the chicken is cooked through and browned on both sides.
6. Serve hot, and enjoy!

To make it a full dinner, you may add additional veggies to the skewers, such as onions, peppers, and cherry tomatoes. Just be sure you adjust the cooking time appropriately.

5.3 Garlic and Herb Roasted Turkey

Garlic and herb roasted turkey is a delightful and savory recipe for a Thanksgiving or holiday turkey. Here's a recipe that you may follow:

Ingredients:

- 1 (12-15 pound) turkey, giblets and neck removed
- 1/2 cup unsalted butter, softened
- 3 tablespoons chopped fresh sage
- 3 tablespoons chopped fresh rosemary

- 3 tablespoons chopped new thyme
- 1 tablespoon garlic powder
- 2 teaspoons salt
- 1 teaspoon freshly ground black pepper
- 1 lemon, halved
- 1 onion, quartered
- 1 head of garlic, halved crosswise
- 2 cups chicken broth

Instructions:

1. Preheat the oven to 325°F (160°C).
2. Rinse the turkey under cold water and blot it dry with paper towels.
3. Add butter, sage, rosemary, thyme, garlic powder, salt, and

black pepper in a small bowl. Mix thoroughly.

4. Gently loosen the turkey's skin by sliding your fingers beneath it. Spread some herb butter below the skin, careful not to rip it.

5. Stuff the bird's cavity with lemon, Onion, and garlic.

6. Tie the legs together with kitchen twine and tuck the wings beneath the bird.

7. Rub the leftover herb butter all over the bird.

8. Place the turkey in a roasting pan and pour the chicken stock into the bottom.

9. Cover the turkey with foil and roast for 2 1/2 to 3 hours, occasionally basting with the pan juices.

10. Remove the foil and continue to roast for another 30 minutes or until the turkey's internal temperature reaches 165°F (74°C).
11. Remove the turkey from the oven and let it rest for 20 minutes before cutting.

Enjoy your wonderful and savory garlic and herb-roasted turkey.

5.4 AIP Shepherd's Pie

Here is a recipe for an AIP (Autoimmune Protocol) Shepherd's Pie:

Ingredients:

- 1 pound ground beef
- 1 large onion, diced
- 2 large carrots, diced
- 2 stalks celery, diced
- 2 cloves garlic, minced
- 1 teaspoon salt
- 1 teaspoon dried thyme
- 1/2 teaspoon dried rosemary
- 1/2 teaspoon dried oregano
- 1/2 teaspoon ground cinnamon
- 1/2 teaspoon ground ginger
- 1/2 teaspoon ground turmeric
- 1/4 cup bone broth or water
- 1 head of cauliflower, chopped into florets
- 2 tablespoons coconut oil
- 1/4 teaspoon garlic powder
- Salt to taste

Instructions:

1. Preheat the oven to 375°F.

2. In a large skillet over medium-high heat, cook the ground beef until browned and cooked. Drain any excess fat and set aside.

3. Add the Onion, carrots, and celery in the same skillet, and cook until the vegetables are tender, about 5-7 minutes. Add the minced garlic, salt, thyme, rosemary, oregano, cinnamon, ginger, and turmeric, and simmer for another 1-2 minutes.

4. Add the cooked ground beef back to the pan with the veggies, and pour in the bone broth or water. Mix everything and let it boil for a few minutes

until the liquid has diminished and the mixture has thickened.

5. Meanwhile, cook the cauliflower florets until they are soft. Drain any excess water, and throw the cauliflower in a food processor along with the coconut oil, garlic powder, and salt. Process till the cauliflower is smooth and resembles mashed potatoes.

6. Pour the ground beef and vegetable mixture into a 9x13 inch baking dish, and distribute the mashed cauliflower evenly on top.

7. Bake the shepherd's pie in the oven for 25-30 minutes or until the mashed cauliflower is gently browned on top.

8. Serve hot, and enjoy!

Note: This recipe is AIP-compliant, but please be careful to double-check all ingredients to verify they are healthy for your unique dietary requirements.

CHAPTER SIX

6.0 Side Dishes on the Autoimmune Protocol

The Autoimmune Protocol (AIP) is a diet that attempts to decrease inflammation and repair the stomach in patients with autoimmune diseases. The diet entails removing potentially inflammatory items, such as grains, dairy, legumes, and processed foods, and concentrating on nutrient-dense foods that assist healing, such as vegetables, fruits, and high-quality protein sources.

Regarding side dishes on the AIP, there are many tasty and healthy alternatives.

6.1 Roasted Brussels Sprouts with Bacon and Apple

Roasted Brussels sprouts with bacon and apple is a tasty and easy-to-make side dish that is excellent for any dinner. Here's an easy formula to follow:

Ingredients:

- 1 pound Brussels sprouts, trimmed and halved
- 2 slices of bacon, chopped
- 1 apple, cored and sliced
- 2 tablespoons olive oil
- Salt & pepper to taste

Instructions:

1. Preheat the oven to 400°F (200°C).
2. In a large dish, mix the Brussels sprouts with olive oil, salt, and pepper until thoroughly coated.
3. Place the Brussels sprouts on a baking sheet in a single layer.
4. Sprinkle the chopped bacon over the Brussels sprouts.
5. Roast the Brussels sprouts and bacon in the oven for 15-20 minutes or until the nodes are soft and the bacon is crispy.
6. Add the sliced apple to the baking sheet and roast for 5-10 minutes, until the apple is slightly caramelized and the Brussels sprouts are golden brown.

Once the meal is done, you may serve it immediately and enjoy the exquisite blend of tastes and textures. This recipe is excellent for helping with roasted meats, such as chicken or beef, and it is sure to be a success with your family and friends.

6.2 Garlic and Herb Mashed Cauliflower

Garlic and herb mashed cauliflower is a delightful and healthful alternative to regular mashed potatoes. Here is a recipe to make it:

Ingredients:

- 1 medium head cauliflower

- 2 garlic cloves, minced
- 2 tablespoons unsalted butter
- 2 tablespoons chopped fresh herbs (such as chives, parsley, or thyme)
- Salt and pepper to taste

Instructions:

1. Cut the cauliflower into tiny florets and remove the core.
2. Steam or boil the cauliflower until it is soft, approximately 8-10 minutes.
3. Drain the cauliflower and return it to the saucepan.
4. Add the minced garlic, butter, and chopped herbs to the saucepan.

5. Use an immersion blender or potato masher to mash the cauliflower until it is smooth.
6. Season with salt and pepper to taste.
7. Serve hot.

This recipe serves 4-6 people as a side dish. You may add additional ingredients to modify the taste, such as grated Parmesan cheese, roasted red pepper, or crumbled bacon. Enjoy!

6.3 Roasted Carrots with Thyme

Roasted carrots with thyme are a tasty and easy side dish that can be created with only a few ingredients. Here's a recipe you may follow:

Ingredients:

- 1 pound carrots, peeled and cut into 1-inch pieces
- 2 tablespoons olive oil
- 1 tablespoon fresh thyme leaves \s* Salt and pepper, to taste

Instructions:

1. Preheat your oven to 400°F (200°C).
2. Add the sliced carrots, olive oil, and fresh thyme leaves to a large dish. Toss the carrots until they are equally covered with the oil and thyme.
3. Season the carrots with salt and pepper to taste.

4. Transfer the carrots to a baking sheet, spreading them out in a single layer.
5. Roast the carrots in the oven for 25-30 minutes or until they are soft and gently browned.
6. Serve the roasted carrots hot, topped with more fresh thyme leaves, if preferred.

Enjoy your tasty and nutritious roasted carrots with thyme!

6.4 AIP Fried Plantains

Here's a simple recipe for AIP (Autoimmune Protocol) Fried Plantains:

Ingredients:

- 2 ripe plantains
- 2 tbsp. coconut oil
- Sea salt to taste

Instructions:

1. Peel the plantains and cut them into thin slices (approximately 1/4 inch thick).
2. Heat the coconut oil in a large pan over medium-high heat.
3. Once the oil is heated, add the plantain slices to the pan and cook for approximately 2-3 minutes on each side or until golden brown.
4. Once the plantains are cooked, take them from the pan and lay

them on a dish lined with paper towels to absorb excess oil.

5. Sprinkle it with sea salt to taste.

Enjoy your AIP fried plantains as a beautiful side dish or snack.

CHAPTER SEVEN

7.0 Desserts on the Autoimmune Protocol

The Autoimmune Protocol (AIP) is a specific diet that seeks to decrease inflammation and encourage healing in patients with autoimmune illnesses. The diet removes numerous items typically linked with inflammation or inflammatory responses, including grains, legumes, dairy, nightshade vegetables, processed foods, and refined sweets.

While the AIP diet might be restricted, many tasty and gratifying sweets can still be eaten while following the protocol.

7.1 Chocolate Coconut Pudding

I discovered a hazardous discovery this week. A finding that requires boiling up a can of coconut milk with a handful of lovely chocolate and a little vanilla (and a few other things) and making the silkiest, dreamiest pudding you may have ever eaten.

Although usually relatively straightforward, puddings may occasionally take work. There's nothing worse than a lumpy or gritty pudding or a pudding that doesn't taste like anything. You won't find any of those things here. I chose coconut milk as a basis since it is so creamy and provides just a bit of coconut flavor without overwhelming the chocolate. I was tempted to incorporate a little coconut essence but was eventually scared it would taste fake and too powerful of coconut. As it is today, it is the ideal balance of rich chocolate taste with coconut. You're going to enjoy it.

I always add a little espresso powder to dark chocolate dishes because it gives a deeper dimension and pulls out those darker cocoa flavors. If you don't have espresso powder at home, it's absolutely optional. As with many sweets where the chocolate is the star, use the most excellent quality you can find or afford. I use

Valrhona cocoa powder, which I realize is a luxury, and Scharffen Berger semisweet chocolate chips because they melt nicely.

INGREDIENTS

- 1 (14-ounce) can of coconut milk, divided
- 1/4 cup sugar
- 1/2 teaspoon salt
- 3 tablespoons cornstarch
- 3 tablespoons cocoa powder
- 1/2 teaspoon espresso powder, optional
- 5 ounces 62% semisweet chocolate, coarsely chopped (I use Scharffen Berger)
- 1 teaspoon vanilla extract

- 1/2 cup coconut flakes, toasted, to garnish

INSTRUCTIONS

1. Shake the can of coconut milk as it might settle. In a medium-sized saucepan, bring half the can of coconut milk, sugar, and salt to a simmer over low heat. Could you not allow it to boil totally?

2. Mix the remaining coconut milk, cornstarch, chocolate powder, and espresso powder in a separate small bowl. \s* Slowly add the cornstarch mixture to the hot pan of coconut milk, stirring vigorously. Keep whisking on low heat until the pudding

nearly reaches a simmer once again and thickens, approximately 2 minutes.

3. Remove the pot from heat. Whisk in the chocolate and vanilla. Keep swirling until the chocolate melts into the pudding and the mixture is smooth and silky.

4. Pour pudding into a separate dish and set it in the refrigerator to cool sufficiently for at least 2 hours. To prevent skin from developing, press plastic wraps up on the surface of the pudding.

5. Serve with a sprinkling of toasted coconut flakes. If covered in an airtight container, the pudding may be refrigerated for up to 4 days. It

will harden up quite a bit after being cooled; give it a nice, solid stir before serving.

7.2 AIP Apple Crumble

This Crockpot AIP Apple Crumble is excellent for a simple holiday dessert. Simple and delicious. Your visitors will only know it's AIP and Paleo!

I don't know about you, but when Thanksgiving and Christmas roll around, I am all about that apple crumble! Pies and cakes are delicious, but crumbles and crisps are where it's at.

Unfortunately, all of these traditional holiday desserts aren't celiac-friendly. And they aren't AIP-friendly. As Thanksgiving is fast-approaching, I've been pondering easy dishes for a full-on AIP-friendly Thanksgiving feast that I can quickly make without my family feeling deprived of a typical Thanksgiving.

First on the schedule is this easy, 5-Ingredient Crockpot Apple Crumble. One of the most remarkable things about this AIP Apple Crumble is that it's baked in the Crockpot for a simple, set-it-and-forget-it dessert that will only take up valuable oven space. And you won't have to attempt to balance creating many recipes at once since you can set this first and then go on to the other meals that demand more hands-on time.

Plus, as you know, I am all about simplicity. Especially when it comes to holiday cuisine. If I don't have to worry about complex recipes, I don't worry about burning one dish while I tend to another.

This AIP Apple Crumble may be prepared, set, and ignored until it is time for dessert. Setting your Crockpot to "warm" when it's done cooking will keep the AIP Apple Crumble at the optimum temperature until everyone's ready for it. No lukewarm dessert for you!
Alright, let's start this Crockpot AIP Apple Crumble cookin'!

How to create this Crockpot AIP Apple Crumble Equipment you'll need

First, you'll need a Crockpot or other slow cooker. It will also work if you have an Instant Pot with a slow cooker feature. Then, you'll need a cutting board, a chef's knife, and a vegetable peeler.

AIP Apple Crumble Ingredients

You may use whatever sort of apple you'd like. I love Granny Smith since they give a slight acidity that I appreciate in sweet sweets. In my view, this AIP Apple Crumble has the ideal amount of sweetness. It's not overly sweet at all, but also not too tart. If you choose another variety of apples, you may need to reduce the quantity of maple syrup you use. Otherwise, it can become overly sweet, especially if you put AIP ice cream or coconut whipped cream on top.

Here's what you'll need:

- 4 Granny Smith apples, peeled, cored and diced
- 1/4 cup maple syrup
- 2 Tbsp cassava flour
- 1 tsp ground cinnamon

For the crumble topping:
- 1 cup cassava flour
- 1/4 cup coconut oil, melted
- 1/4 tsp ground cinnamon

Instructions

Peel, core, and dice your apples and add them to the Crockpot. Add the maple syrup, 2 Tbsp cassava flour, and 1 tsp ground cinnamon to the saucepan and mix to cover the apples evenly.

Add the crumble topping ingredients to a small mixing dish and swirl to incorporate. The mixture will be crumbly. Sprinkle over the diced apples.

Can I double the recipe?

Absolutely! There's enough space left in the Crockpot to double this recipe, but I have yet to try it.

Double the recipe and add half an hour to the cooking time to account for the added volume.

How do I keep the leftovers?

Any leftovers you have of this AIP Apple Crumble may be kept in an airtight jar in the fridge for up to three days. I split myself up into serving-size mason jars, for convenient post-Thanksgiving goodies. To reheat, throw in the microwave for about a minute, or heat in an oven or toaster oven at 350ºF for a few minutes. Make sure your container is oven and microwave-safe. You may also have the leftovers cold, straight out of the fridge, but I prefer them better when they're warm.

7.3 AIP Pumpkin Pie

This Grain-free Pumpkin Pie features a light and flaky crust that you'll never believe is AIP and paleo. The filling is thick and aromatic with all your favorite pumpkin spices and is dairy and coconut free.

Confession: I'm not a pumpkin pie lover! I didn't grow up with it and simply don't really appreciate the taste of canned pumpkin puree, but so many of you wanted a paleo and AIP Pumpkin Pie so here it is! My spouse, who particularly loves pumpkin pie, has given this recipe excellent ratings, so I hope you like it!

Unlike other paleo pumpkin pies, this AIP-compliant dish is egg-free, nut-free, coconut-free, and allergy-friendly. This healthy version is RICH in flavor and doesn't sacrifice texture!

While the crust is cooked, the filling is simply refrigerated in the fridge to firm. The nut-free crust on this pie is absolutely excellent. The trick to nailing it is to ensure the palm shortening is completely frozen before you begin working with it and to work quickly so as not to warm it up too much before it bakes in the oven.

HERE ARE THE KEY INGREDIENTS IN THIS AIP/PALEO PUMPKIN PIE:

For the Easy, Homemade, No-bake Pumpkin Pie Filling, you'll need the following:

- pumpkin puree – I use canned pumpkin puree for this recipe. Make sure it's nice and smooth before you begin to bake. I prefer to whip mine in a food processor or blender.
- Maple syrup – the unrefined sweetener in this filling
- Tapioca starch – this helps thicken the pumpkin pie filling without eggs or dairy
- Cinnamon and powdered ginger – these warm spices

produce that iconic pumpkin pie flavor

- Gelatin – this is necessary for the pie filling to set For the Grain-free, Nut-free Pie Crust, you'll need
- Palm shortening – not palm oil! It would help if you had palm shortening in this recipe that you freeze before baking.
- Cassava flour – I recommend Bob's Red Mill or Otto's in this recipe. Making this AIP/paleo pumpkin pie with cassava flour keeps this recipe grain-free, gluten-free, nut-free, and allergy-friendly.
- Coconut or maple sugar – use maple sugar if you want the crust to have a lighter color or if you cannot tolerate coconut

- Apple cider vinegar and ice cold water – the vinegar is used to tenderize the dough, and the ice cold water keeps the shortening cold and binds the dough together

CAN I MAKE A PALEO PUMPKIN PIE WITHOUT EGGS?

Yes! This egg-free AIP pumpkin pie recipe utilizes gelatin as a binder and tapioca starch to thicken the pie filling.

WHAT SIZE PIE DOES THIS RECIPE MAKE?

One regular 9-inch pie.

IS THERE A SUBSTITUTE FOR THE PALM SHORTENING IN THIS GRAIN-FREE PIE CRUST?

If you can't find palm shortening where you live, replace it with an alternative gluten-free pastry crust here. I have 4 distinct varieties, which are all dairy-free, egg-free, and nut-free! Check them out in our article on How to Make Grain-Free Pie Crust.

WHAT DO YOU SERVE WITH AIP/PALEO PUMPKIN PIE?

This pie is excellent with whipped cream or coconut-based ice cream if you can tolerate coconut.

HOW DO I STORE THIS DAIRY-FREE, GLUTEN-FREE AIP PUMPKIN PIE?

Store in the fridge in a sealed container or the pie dish wrapped. Bring to room temperature before serving. I don't advocate reheating this pie since the gelatin will lose its grip.

7.4 Coconut Milk Ice Cream

This delicious coconut ice cream recipe is a vegan and dairy-free treat you can prepare at home, with no ice cream machine necessary!

You can create this coconut ice cream with only FOUR ingredients:

Vanilla extract
Sweetener of choice
A pinch of salt

In only a few simple steps and with many various flavor possibilities, a luscious bowl of creamy handmade coconut milk ice cream may be all yours!

Chocolate Coconut Ice Cream

To make the vanilla version below into chocolate coconut milk ice cream instead, add one-fourth cup of cocoa powder at the beginning.

Or create Nutella coconut ice cream by combining three to four tablespoons of chocolate hazelnut spread or this Homemade Nutella Recipe into the chocolate base.

You may use standard unsweetened cocoa powder, Dutch process cocoa, raw cacao powder, or powdered hot chocolate mix for the chocolate ice cream.

Coconut Ice Cream Flavors

- Coffee Ice Cream: Use the basic coconut ice cream recipe below. Add two tablespoons of regular or decaf instant coffee to the liquid ingredients.

- Peanut Butter Ice Cream: Stir one-fourth cup of peanut butter into the liquid ingredients, then add some micro chocolate chips as desired.

- Cookie Dough Ice Cream: Use the regular ice cream recipe. Stir in small spoonfuls of this Chickpea Cookie Dough Dip or bits of your favorite eggless cookie dough (or the dough from any of my healthy cookie recipes) into the ice cream after mixing.

- Strawberry Ice Cream: Add one cup of strawberries, stems removed, to the basic recipe before mixing. Omit the additional half-cup milk of choice.

- Salted Caramel Ice Cream: Swirl in homemade Coconut Caramel and add a quick sprinkling of sea salt and shaved chocolate, if preferred, to the top of each serving.

How to utilize a can of coconut milk

Canned coconut milk is one of my favorite items to utilize in recipes.
It is an excellent alternative for heavy cream in sweet and savory foods such as smoothies, milkshakes, pies, puddings, soups, or curries.

You may cook Coconut Curry or my handmade Chocolate Truffles.
You may use it for Coconut Whipped Cream. Or you can even substitute coconut milk instead of cow's milk for this reader's favorite dessert recipe for Chocolate Banana Bread.

Especially with studies identifying over 60-75% of the world's population as lactose intolerant, we will start to see more and more items on the market being created with coconut milk instead of dairy in the following years.

Can you create ice cream using coconut milk?

Yes, you indeed can! If you have dairy allergies, are vegan, or even want to try something new and delicious, coconut milk is the ideal ingredient to produce rich and creamy ice cream without any natural cream.

Many prominent companies, such as Haagen Dazs, So Delicious, Ben & Jerry's, and Halo Top, are even hopping on the dairy-free coconut ice cream bandwagon.

However, by creating your ice cream at home, you choose what ingredients go in (less sugar and no corn syrup, gums, or preservatives) and also select what flavors to produce.

Recipe tips and techniques

Be careful to use whole-fat canned coconut milk for the recipe, not light coconut milk.

And do not replace a carton of chilled coconut milk beverage, since this is not the same product and needs to contain more fat to make velvety ice cream.

Culinary coconut milk generally comes in a can. Some popular brands of coconut milk are Thai Kitchen, Whole Foods, Goya, Chaokoh, and Native Forest.
Due to the absence of preservatives and gums, handmade ice cream is best the day it is created. This is

when it will have the creamiest
texture.

CHAPTER EIGHT

8.0 Tips for Sticking to the Autoimmune Protocol

Suppose most of us start on the Autoimmune Protocol (AIP) template believing we'll give it a red-hot try for a time and then – when we feel better – we'll be able to return to our old way of living…

Our previous way of life is precisely what got us into this situation in the first place. This is why we must tailor our own AIP way of life for the long run — alter the template to match our demands over time.

Unfortunately, just because we learn to realize this as our new reality doesn't mean our AIP way of life becomes a stroll in the park!

No matter how seasoned you are at your healing protocol, there are times when life gets in the way, and your AIP wheels might go shaky, whether it's the food, lifestyle factors, or both.

I've been following my AIP lifestyle for about 5 years now.

HERE ARE MY 5 TOP TIPS FOR (RE)FINDING YOUR AIP GROOVE:

8.1 TAKE IT BACK TO BASICS

The program is an elimination diet to repair the gut. Focusing on nutritional density (bone broth, leafy greens, 8-12 cups veggies per day, liver, shellfish) to flood out food choices that aren't benefiting you is a fantastic strategy to get back on track.

If you're out of the habit of maintaining a food and mood journal, now's the time to start that again - it's the most excellent method to keep yourself honest!

8.2 CREATE RITUALS THAT WORK FOR YOU

For any regimen to function long-term, we must build habits that suit our lifestyle. This involves finding tools and tactics that both simplify and customize your procedure.

Three things genuinely made a difference for me:

- Develop a morning routine, a series of behaviors unique to you (that don't entail checking in with social media!) to help get you off on the right foot for the day. My morning routine involves a stroll with my dog facing the rising light, a few simple yoga postures, and establishing a goal for my day.

- If sleep is difficult, why not work on your own personal 'Operation Sleepy Time'? Our body recovers while we are sleeping. Creating a nighttime routine to allow your body every chance to enjoy great, peaceful sleep helps boost healing and aid with handling life's curve balls.

- Create a recipe folder for your 'regular favorites.' These are the tried and true dishes you and your family enjoy and that you know work every time. Having the folder on hand reduces some of the tension of what to prepare on evenings when you've lost your culinary mojo. (Sophie's No Nightshade

Ratatouille is featured in my folder!)

8.3 ACCEPT THAT YOU ARE HUMAN

"Compassion involves complete absorption in the state of being human." – Henri Nouwen.

In my coaching business, I assist those suffering from chronic disease utilizing the AIP template as a basis for food and lifestyle transformation. One of the most continuously harsh elements for many of my clients is cultivating self-compassion. We have the propensity to be difficult on ourselves and hold ourselves to a higher standard than others.

The problem is – you are human. You will slip up. Everyone does, and that is fine. Any form of therapeutic procedure may be tough to manage. The crucial thing is that you be kind to yourself when this occurs, and – at the same time – that you concentrate on building the self-awareness to understand precisely why or how the mistake happened; if this is a habit you feel needs correction, and what you're going to do about it.

Hint: if you're serious about developing your self-compassion muscle, try building a regular 'loving kindness' meditation into your mindfulness routine.

8.4 IT'S NOT JUST ABOUT DIET

When we start out on AIP, it's easy to think that it's all about diet. Our diet can be the most nutrient-dense approach, but if we fail to address poor lifestyle habits, chances are our health will not improve. Lifestyle habits matter.

Factoring in things like sleep, stress management, connection, getting outside, and moving... all have a part to play in healing.

8.5 GET SOME SUPPORT

Social isolation is on the increase. But did you know there is an increasing association between social isolation and people who suffer from chronic disease?

You could be the most dyed-in-the-wool introvert, yet you still need human interaction and support to survive.

This AIP way of life might be brutal to traverse on your own. It helps to locate folks who understand. It's one of the primary reasons I designed the 30-day AIP Reset (use code SOPHIE for 15% OFF). There are fantastic resources for individuals starting on AIP, but they are not so accessible to veteran AIPers trying to keep on track or recalibrate…

Back in August 2016, I needed to reassess my AIP efforts. My AIP wheels were shaky! I expressed my desire to have a Reset to several of my readers, and a few of them indicated they would want to join me. Before shortly, we had 127 seasoned AIPers performing a Reset together. The support and companionship were fantastic.